without

Crash

Diet

and

Gym

Food Diary

Anne Bauer

ISBN-10: 1507585578
ISBN-13: 978-1507585573

DEDICATION

This book is dedicated to all people who are dissatisfied with their bodies and want to do something about it.

You already made the first step on your way – now you just need to keep on walking. I know you can make it as long as you don't give up!

Together with the knowledge of the book *'Without Crash Diet and Gym: my secret to achieve this body'* this food diary should help you to recognize and improve your eating habits in order to form your dream body. For more information check the author's website: **www.4thebetteryou.wordpress.com**.

Good Luck!

EXPLANATION

If you want to lose weight then one of the most important things to begin with is to note down what you are eating and when. This is the only way to recognize why you carry too much weight. Besides, in order to change your old eating habits and adapt to your new ones, it is essential to document what and when you eat and drink. Thus you can identify your progress as well as areas in need of further improvement.

This food diary is designed to help you documenting these exact things so you can keep track and change for the better. At the very beginning of the journal, as well as after 4 and 8 weeks, you will find the Appraisal. It should be used to determine your bench mark data and to keep record of your improved data (after 4 and 8 weeks). Within the rest of the pages you should document your nutrition each day for 2 months. Mostly, those 2 months of documentation are sufficient to

1. Find the 'defect' in your nutrition.
2. Improve your nutrition.
3. Get used to your changed nutrition.

After 2 months it is very likely that you won't need the documentation anymore. Nevertheless, in case you prefer to keep track of your nutrition you now already have a good draft of a food diary with this book.

APPRAISAL

Date:_____

Weight:_____

Body Fat:_____

Circumference
Tight:_____

Hip:_____

Waist:_____

Upper Arm:_____

Total Daily Energy Expenditure:_____
Daily Energy Intake:_____

Things I like about my body:

1._____

2._____

3._____

_____

Things I dislike about my body:

1._____

2._____

3._____

_____

Things I want to change:

1._____

2._____

3._____

_____

What is the reason for my weight?

_____

_____

FOOD DIARY

MONDAY   Date:_____

Breakfast: Time:_____

ate:_____

_____

_____

drank:_____

_____

Protein:_____ Fat:_____

Carbohydrate:_____

Snack: Time:_____

_____

_____

_____

Lunch: Time:_____

ate:_____

_____

_____

drank:_____

_____

Protein:_____ Fat:_____

Carbohydrate:_____

Snack: Time:_____

_____

_____

_____

Dinner: Time:_____

ate:_____

_____

_____

drank:_____

_____

Protein:_____ Fat:_____

Carbohydrate:_____

Daily Energy Intake:_____

Notes:_____

TUESDAY   Date:_____

Breakfast: Time:_____

ate:_____

_____

_____

drank:_____

_____

Protein:_____ Fat:_____

Carbohydrate:_____

Snack: Time:_____

_____

_____

_____

Lunch: Time:_____

ate:_____

_____

_____

drank:_____

_____

Protein:_____ Fat:_____

Carbohydrate:_____

<u>Snack:</u>   Time:_____

_____

_____

_____

<u>Dinner:</u>   Time:_____

ate:_____

_____

_____

drank:_____

_____

Protein:_____ Fat:_____

Carbohydrate:_____

<u>Daily Energy Intake:</u>_____

Notes:_____

_____

_____

WEDNESDAY

Date:_____

Breakfast:

Time:_____

ate:_____

_____

_____

drank:_____

_____

Protein:_____ Fat:_____

Carbohydrate:_____

Snack:

Time:_____

_____

_____

_____

Lunch:

Time:_____

ate:_____

_____

_____

drank:_____

_____

Protein:_____ Fat:_____

Carbohydrate:_____

<u>Snack:</u>   Time:_____

_____

_____

_____

<u>Dinner:</u>   Time:_____

ate:_____

_____

_____

drank:_____

_____

Protein:_____ Fat:_____

Carbohydrate:_____

<u>Daily Energy Intake:</u>_____

Notes:_____

_____

_____

THURSDAY

Date:_____

Breakfast:

Time:_____

ate:_____

_____

_____

drank:_____

_____

Protein:_____ Fat:_____

Carbohydrate:_____

Snack:

Time:_____

_____

_____

_____

Lunch:

Time:_____

ate:_____

_____

_____

drank:_____

_____

Protein:_____ Fat:_____

Carbohydrate:_____

Snack: Time:_____

_____

_____

_____

Dinner: Time:_____

ate:_____

_____

_____

drank:_____

_____

Protein:_____ Fat:_____

Carbohydrate:_____

<u>Daily Energy Intake:</u>_____

Notes:_____

_____

_____

FRIDAY   Date:_____

Breakfast: Time:_____

ate:_____

_____

_____

drank:_____

_____

Protein:_____ Fat:_____

Carbohydrate:_____

Snack: Time:_____

_____

_____

_____

Lunch: Time:_____

ate:_____

_____

_____

drank:_____

_____

Protein:_____ Fat:_____

Carbohydrate:_____

<u>Snack:</u>   Time:_____

_____

_____

_____

<u>Dinner:</u>   Time:_____

ate:_____

_____

_____

drank:_____

_____

Protein:_____ Fat:_____

Carbohydrate:_____

<u>Daily Energy Intake:</u>_____

Notes:_____

_____

_____

SATURDAY   Date:_____

Breakfast: Time:_____

ate:_____

_____

_____

drank:_____

_____

Protein:_____ Fat:_____

Carbohydrate:_____

Snack: Time:_____

_____

_____

_____

Lunch: Time:_____

ate:_____

_____

_____

drank:_____

_____

Protein:_____ Fat:_____

Carbohydrate:_____

Snack: Time:_____

_____

_____

_____

Dinner: Time:_____

ate:_____

_____

_____

drank:_____

_____

Protein:_____ Fat:_____

Carbohydrate:_____

<u>Daily Energy Intake:</u>_____

Notes:_____

_____

_____

SUNDAY   Date:_____

Breakfast: Time:_____

ate:_____

_____

_____

drank:_____

_____

Protein:_____ Fat:_____

Carbohydrate:_____

Snack: Time:_____

_____

_____

_____

Lunch: Time:_____

ate:_____

_____

_____

drank:_____

_____

Protein:_____ Fat:_____

Carbohydrate:_____

<u>Snack:</u>   Time:_____

_____

_____

_____

<u>Dinner:</u>   Time:_____

ate:_____

_____

_____

drank:_____

_____

Protein:_____ Fat:_____

Carbohydrate:_____

<u>Daily Energy Intake:</u>_____

Notes:_____

_____

_____

MONDAY

Date:_____

Breakfast:

Time:_____

ate:_____

_____

_____

drank:_____

_____

Protein:_____ Fat:_____

Carbohydrate:_____

Snack:

Time:_____

_____

_____

_____

Lunch:

Time:_____

ate:_____

_____

_____

drank:_____

_____

Protein:_____ Fat:_____

Carbohydrate:_____

Snack: Time:_____

_____

_____

_____

Dinner: Time:_____

ate:_____

_____

_____

drank:_____

_____

Protein:_____ Fat:_____

Carbohydrate:_____

Daily Energy Intake:_____

Notes:_____

_____

_____

TUESDAY   Date:_____

Breakfast: Time:_____

ate:_____

_____

_____

drank:_____

_____

Protein:_____ Fat:_____

Carbohydrate:_____

Snack: Time:_____

_____

_____

_____

Lunch: Time:_____

ate:_____

_____

_____

drank:_____

_____

Protein:_____ Fat:_____

Carbohydrate:_____

Snack: Time:_____

_____

_____

_____

Dinner: Time:_____

ate:_____

_____

_____

drank:_____

_____

Protein:_____ Fat:_____

Carbohydrate:_____

<u>Daily Energy Intake:</u>_____

Notes:_____

_____

_____

WEDNESDAY

Date:_____

Breakfast:

Time:_____

ate:_____

_____

_____

drank:_____

_____

Protein:_____ Fat:_____

Carbohydrate:_____

Snack:

Time:_____

_____

_____

_____

Lunch:

Time:_____

ate:_____

_____

_____

drank:_____

_____

Protein:_____ Fat:_____

Carbohydrate:_____

Snack: Time:_____

_____

_____

_____

Dinner: Time:_____

ate:_____

_____

_____

drank:_____

_____

Protein:_____ Fat:_____

Carbohydrate:_____

Daily Energy Intake:_____

Notes:_____

_____

_____

THURSDAY   Date:_____

Breakfast: Time:_____

ate:_____

_____

_____

drank:_____

_____

Protein:_____ Fat:_____

Carbohydrate:_____

Snack: Time:_____

_____

_____

_____

Lunch: Time:_____

ate:_____

_____

_____

drank:_____

_____

Protein:_____ Fat:_____

Carbohydrate:_____

<u>Snack:</u>   Time:_____

_____

_____

_____

<u>Dinner:</u>   Time:_____

ate:_____

_____

_____

drank:_____

_____

Protein:_____ Fat:_____

Carbohydrate:_____

<u>Daily Energy Intake:</u>_____

Notes:_____

_____

_____

FRIDAY   Date:_____

Breakfast: Time:_____

ate:_____

_____

_____

drank:_____

_____

Protein:_____ Fat:_____

Carbohydrate:_____

Snack: Time:_____

_____

_____

_____

Lunch: Time:_____

ate:_____

_____

_____

drank:_____

_____

Protein:_____ Fat:_____

Carbohydrate:_____

Snack: Time:_____

_____

_____

_____

Dinner: Time:_____

ate:_____

_____

drank:_____

Protein:_____ Fat:_____

Carbohydrate:_____

Daily Energy Intake:_____

Notes:_____

_____

_____

SATURDAY   Date:_____

Breakfast: Time:_____

ate:_____

_____

_____

drank:_____

_____

Protein:_____ Fat:_____

Carbohydrate:_____

Snack: Time:_____

_____

_____

_____

Lunch: Time:_____

ate:_____

_____

_____

drank:_____

_____

Protein:_____ Fat:_____
Carbohydrate:_____

Snack: Time:_____

_____
_____
_____

Dinner: Time:_____
ate:_____
_____
_____
drank:_____
_____
Protein:_____ Fat:_____
Carbohydrate:_____

<u>Daily Energy Intake:</u>_____
Notes:_____
_____
_____

SUNDAY   Date:_____

Breakfast: Time:_____

ate:_____

_____

_____

drank:_____

_____

Protein:_____ Fat:_____

Carbohydrate:_____

Snack: Time:_____

_____

_____

_____

Lunch: Time:_____

ate:_____

_____

_____

drank:_____

_____

Protein:_____ Fat:_____

Carbohydrate:_____

Snack: Time:_____

_____

_____

_____

Dinner: Time:_____

ate:_____

_____

_____

drank:_____

_____

Protein:_____ Fat:_____

Carbohydrate:_____

<u>Daily Energy Intake:</u>_____

Notes:_____

_____

_____

MONDAY   Date:_____

Breakfast: Time:_____

ate:_____

_____

_____

drank:_____

_____

Protein:_____ Fat:_____

Carbohydrate:_____

Snack: Time:_____

_____

_____

_____

Lunch: Time:_____

ate:_____

_____

_____

drank:_____

_____

Protein:_____ Fat:_____

Carbohydrate:_____

<u>Snack:</u> Time:_____

_____

_____

_____

<u>Dinner:</u> Time:_____

ate:_____

_____

_____

drank:_____

_____

Protein:_____ Fat:_____

Carbohydrate:_____

<u>Daily Energy Intake:</u>_____

Notes:_____

_____

_____

TUESDAY   Date:_____

Breakfast: Time:_____

ate:_____

_____

_____

drank:_____

_____

Protein:_____ Fat:_____

Carbohydrate:_____

Snack: Time:_____

_____

_____

_____

Lunch: Time:_____

ate:_____

_____

_____

drank:_____

_____

Protein:_____ Fat:_____

Carbohydrate:_____

Snack: Time:_____

_____

_____

_____

Dinner: Time:_____

ate:_____

_____

_____

drank:_____

_____

Protein:_____ Fat:_____

Carbohydrate:_____

<u>Daily Energy Intake:</u>_____

Notes:_____

_____

_____

WEDNESDAY Date:_____

Breakfast: Time:_____

ate:_____

_____

_____

drank:_____

_____

Protein:_____ Fat:_____

Carbohydrate:_____

Snack: Time:_____

_____

_____

_____

Lunch: Time:_____

ate:_____

_____

_____

drank:_____

_____

Protein:_____ Fat:_____

Carbohydrate:_____

<u>Snack:</u>   Time:_____

_____

_____

_____

<u>Dinner:</u>   Time:_____

ate:_____

_____

_____

drank:_____

_____

Protein:_____ Fat:_____

Carbohydrate:_____

<u>Daily Energy Intake:</u>_____

Notes:_____

_____

_____

THURSDAY

Date:_____

Breakfast:

Time:_____

ate:_____

_____

_____

drank:_____

_____

Protein:_____ Fat:_____

Carbohydrate:_____

Snack:

Time:_____

_____

_____

_____

Lunch:

Time:_____

ate:_____

_____

_____

drank:_____

_____

Protein:_____ Fat:_____

Carbohydrate:_____

Snack: Time:_____

_____

_____

_____

Dinner: Time:_____

ate:_____

_____

_____

drank:_____

_____

Protein:_____ Fat:_____

Carbohydrate:_____

Daily Energy Intake:_____

Notes:_____

_____

_____

FRIDAY Date:_____

Breakfast: Time:_____

ate:_____

_____

_____

drank:_____

_____

Protein:_____ Fat:_____

Carbohydrate:_____

Snack: Time:_____

_____

_____

_____

Lunch: Time:_____

ate:_____

_____

_____

drank:_____

_____

Protein:_____ Fat:_____

Carbohydrate:_____

Snack: Time:_____

_____

_____

_____

Dinner: Time:_____

ate:_____

_____

_____

drank:_____

_____

Protein:_____ Fat:_____

Carbohydrate:_____

Daily Energy Intake:_____

Notes:_____

_____

_____

SATURDAY   Date:_____

Breakfast: Time:_____

ate:_____

_____

_____

drank:_____

_____

Protein:_____ Fat:_____

Carbohydrate:_____

Snack: Time:_____

_____

_____

_____

Lunch: Time:_____

ate:_____

_____

_____

drank:_____

_____

Protein:_____ Fat:_____

Carbohydrate:_____

<u>Snack:</u>   Time:_____

_____

_____

_____

<u>Dinner:</u>   Time:_____

ate:_____

_____

_____

drank:_____

_____

Protein:_____ Fat:_____

Carbohydrate:_____

<u>Daily Energy Intake:</u>_____

Notes:_____

_____

_____

SUNDAY   Date:_____

Breakfast: Time:_____

ate:_____

_____

_____

drank:_____

_____

Protein:_____ Fat:_____

Carbohydrate:_____

Snack: Time:_____

_____

_____

_____

Lunch: Time:_____

ate:_____

_____

_____

drank:_____

_____

Protein:_____ Fat:_____

Carbohydrate:_____

Snack: Time:_____

_____

_____

_____

Dinner: Time:_____

ate:_____

_____

_____

drank:_____

_____

Protein:_____ Fat:_____

Carbohydrate:_____

Daily Energy Intake:_____

Notes:_____

_____

_____

MONDAY   Date:_____

Breakfast: Time:_____

ate:_____

_____

_____

drank:_____

_____

Protein:_____ Fat:_____

Carbohydrate:_____

Snack: Time:_____

_____

_____

_____

Lunch: Time:_____

ate:_____

_____

_____

drank:_____

_____

Protein:_____ Fat:_____

Carbohydrate:_____

Snack: Time:_____

_____

_____

_____

Dinner: Time:_____

ate:_____

_____

_____

drank:_____

_____

Protein:_____ Fat:_____

Carbohydrate:_____

Daily Energy Intake:_____

Notes:_____

_____

_____

TUESDAY   Date:_____

Breakfast: Time:_____

ate:_____

_____

_____

drank:_____

_____

Protein:_____ Fat:_____

Carbohydrate:_____

Snack: Time:_____

_____

_____

_____

Lunch: Time:_____

ate:_____

_____

_____

drank:_____

_____

Protein:_____ Fat:_____

Carbohydrate:_____

<u>Snack:</u>   Time:_____

_____

_____

_____

<u>Dinner:</u>   Time:_____

ate:_____

_____

_____

drank:_____

_____

Protein:_____ Fat:_____

Carbohydrate:_____

<u>Daily Energy Intake:</u> ·_____

Notes:_____

_____

_____

WEDNESDAY   Date:_____

<u>**Breakfast:**</u>   Time:_____

ate:_____

_____

_____

drank:_____

_____

Protein:_____ Fat:_____

Carbohydrate:_____

<u>**Snack:**</u>   Time:_____

_____

_____

_____

<u>**Lunch:**</u>   Time:_____

ate:_____

_____

_____

drank:_____

_____

Protein:_____ Fat:_____

Carbohydrate:_____

<u>Snack:</u>   Time:_____

_____

_____

_____

<u>Dinner:</u>   Time:_____

ate:_____

_____

_____

drank:_____

_____

Protein:_____ Fat:_____

Carbohydrate:_____

<u>Daily Energy Intake:</u>_____

Notes:_____

_____

_____

THURSDAY
Date:_____

Breakfast:
Time:_____

ate:_____

_____

_____

drank:_____

_____

Protein:_____ Fat:_____

Carbohydrate:_____

Snack:
Time:_____

_____

_____

_____

Lunch:
Time:_____

ate:_____

_____

_____

drank:_____

_____

Protein:_____ Fat:_____

Carbohydrate:_____

<u>Snack:</u>   Time:_____

_____

_____

_____

<u>Dinner:</u>   Time:_____

ate:_____

_____

_____

drank:_____

_____

Protein:_____ Fat:_____

Carbohydrate:_____

<u>Daily Energy Intake:</u>_____

Notes:_____

_____

_____

FRIDAY   Date:_____

Breakfast: Time:_____

ate:_____

_____

_____

drank:_____

_____

Protein:_____ Fat:_____

Carbohydrate:_____

Snack: Time:_____

_____

_____

_____

Lunch: Time:_____

ate:_____

_____

_____

drank:_____

_____

Protein:_____ Fat:_____

Carbohydrate:_____

Snack: Time:_____

_____

_____

_____

Dinner: Time:_____

ate:_____

_____

_____

drank:_____

_____

Protein:_____ Fat:_____

Carbohydrate:_____

Daily Energy Intake:_____

Notes:_____

_____

_____

SATURDAY   Date:_____

Breakfast: Time:_____

ate:_____

_____

_____

drank:_____

_____

Protein:_____ Fat:_____

Carbohydrate:_____

Snack: Time:_____

_____

_____

_____

Lunch: Time:_____

ate:_____

_____

_____

drank:_____

_____

Protein:_____ Fat:_____

Carbohydrate:_____

Snack: Time:_____

_____

_____

_____

Dinner: Time:_____

ate:_____

_____

_____

drank:_____

_____

Protein:_____ Fat:_____

Carbohydrate:_____

Daily Energy Intake:_____

Notes:_____

_____

_____

SUNDAY Date:_____

Breakfast: Time:_____

ate:_____

_____

_____

drank:_____

_____

Protein:_____ Fat:_____

Carbohydrate:_____

Snack: Time:_____

_____

_____

_____

Lunch: Time:_____

ate:_____

_____

_____

drank:_____

_____

Protein:_____ Fat:_____

Carbohydrate:_____

Snack: Time:_____

_____

_____

_____

Dinner: Time:_____

ate:_____

_____

_____

drank:_____

_____

Protein:_____ Fat:_____

Carbohydrate:_____

Daily Energy Intake:_____

Notes:_____

_____

_____

APPRAISAL

Date:_____

Weight:
at the beginning_____ now _____

Body Fat:
at the beginning_____ now _____

Circumference
Tight:
at the beginning_____ now _____

Hip:
at the beginning_____ now _____

Waist:
at the beginning_____ now _____

Upper Arm:
at the beginning_____ now _____

Total Daily Energy Expenditure:_____
Daily Energy Intake:_____

Things about my body that already changed:

1._____

2._____

3._____

_____

_____

Things about my nutrition that already changed:

1._____

2._____

3._____

_____

_____

Things I still want to change:

1._____

2._____

3._____

_____

_____

MONDAY

Date:_____

Breakfast:

Time:_____

ate:_____

_____

_____

drank:_____

_____

Protein:_____ Fat:_____

Carbohydrate:_____

Snack:

Time:_____

_____

_____

_____

Lunch:

Time:_____

ate:_____

_____

_____

drank:_____

_____

Protein:_____ Fat:_____

Carbohydrate:_____

Snack: Time:_____

_____

_____

_____

Dinner: Time:_____

ate:_____

_____

_____

drank:_____

_____

Protein:_____ Fat:_____

Carbohydrate:_____

Daily Energy Intake:_____

Notes:_____

_____

_____

TUESDAY

Date:_____

Breakfast:

Time:_____

ate:_____

_____

_____

drank:_____

_____

Protein:_____ Fat:_____

Carbohydrate:_____

Snack:

Time:_____

_____

_____

_____

Lunch:

Time:_____

ate:_____

_____

_____

drank:_____

_____

Protein:_____ Fat:_____

Carbohydrate:_____

Snack: Time:_____

_____

_____

_____

Dinner: Time:_____

ate:_____

_____

_____

drank:_____

_____

Protein:_____ Fat:_____

Carbohydrate:_____

<u>Daily Energy Intake:</u>_____

Notes:_____

_____

_____

WEDNESDAY

Date:_____

Breakfast:

Time:_____

ate:_____

_____

_____

drank:_____

_____

Protein:_____ Fat:_____

Carbohydrate:_____

Snack:

Time:_____

_____

_____

_____

Lunch:

Time:_____

ate:_____

_____

_____

drank:_____

_____

Protein:_____ Fat:_____

Carbohydrate:_____

<u>Snack:</u>   Time:_____

_____

_____

_____

<u>Dinner:</u>   Time:_____

ate:_____

_____

_____

drank:_____

_____

Protein:_____ Fat:_____

Carbohydrate:_____

<u>Daily Energy Intake:</u>_____

Notes:_____

_____

_____

THURSDAY   Date:_____

Breakfast: Time:_____

ate:_____

_____

_____

drank:_____

_____

Protein:_____ Fat:_____

Carbohydrate:_____

Snack: Time:_____

_____

_____

_____

Lunch: Time:_____

ate:_____

_____

_____

drank:_____

_____

Protein:_____ Fat:_____

Carbohydrate:_____

Snack: Time:_____

_____

_____

_____

Dinner: Time:_____

ate:_____

_____

_____

drank:_____

_____

Protein:_____ Fat:_____

Carbohydrate:_____

<u>Daily Energy Intake:</u>_____

Notes:_____

_____

_____

FRIDAY Date:_____

Breakfast: Time:_____

ate:_____

_____

_____

drank:_____

_____

Protein:_____ Fat:_____

Carbohydrate:_____

Snack: Time:_____

_____

_____

_____

Lunch: Time:_____

ate:_____

_____

_____

drank:_____

_____

Protein:_____ Fat:_____

Carbohydrate:_____

Snack: Time:_____

_____

_____

_____

Dinner: Time:_____

ate:_____

_____

_____

drank:_____

_____

Protein:_____ Fat:_____

Carbohydrate:_____

Daily Energy Intake:_____

Notes:_____

_____

_____

SATURDAY   Date:_____

Breakfast: Time:_____

ate:_____

_____

_____

drank:_____

_____

Protein:_____ Fat:_____

Carbohydrate:_____

Snack: Time:_____

_____

_____

_____

Lunch: Time:_____

ate:_____

_____

_____

drank:_____

_____

Protein:_____ Fat:_____

Carbohydrate:_____

<u>Snack:</u>   Time:_____

_____

_____

_____

<u>Dinner:</u>   Time:_____

ate:_____

_____

_____

drank:_____

_____

Protein:_____ Fat:_____

Carbohydrate:_____

<u>Daily Energy Intake:</u>_____

Notes:_____

_____

_____

SUNDAY   Date:_____

Breakfast: Time:_____

ate:_____

_____

_____

drank:_____

_____

Protein:_____ Fat:_____

Carbohydrate:_____

Snack: Time:_____

_____

_____

_____

Lunch: Time:_____

ate:_____

_____

_____

drank:_____

_____

Protein:_____ Fat:_____

Carbohydrate:_____

<u>Snack:</u> Time:_____

_____

_____

_____

<u>Dinner:</u> Time:_____

ate:_____

_____

_____

drank:_____

_____

Protein:_____ Fat:_____

Carbohydrate:_____

<u>Daily Energy Intake:</u>_____

Notes:_____

_____

_____

MONDAY

Date:_____

Breakfast:

Time:_____

ate:_____

_____

_____

drank:_____

_____

Protein:_____ Fat:_____

Carbohydrate:_____

Snack:

Time:_____

_____

_____

_____

Lunch:

Time:_____

ate:_____

_____

_____

drank:_____

_____

Protein:_____ Fat:_____

Carbohydrate:_____

Snack: Time:_____

_____

_____

_____

Dinner: Time:_____

ate:_____

_____

_____

drank:_____

_____

Protein:_____ Fat:_____

Carbohydrate:_____

Daily Energy Intake:_____

Notes:_____

_____

_____

TUESDAY   Date:_____

Breakfast: Time:_____

ate:_____

_____

_____

drank:_____

_____

Protein:_____ Fat:_____

Carbohydrate:_____

Snack: Time:_____

_____

_____

_____

Lunch: Time:_____

ate:_____

_____

_____

drank:_____

_____

Protein:_____ Fat:_____

Carbohydrate:_____

<u>Snack:</u> Time:_____

_____

_____

_____

<u>Dinner:</u> Time:_____

ate:_____

_____

_____

drank:_____

_____

Protein:_____ Fat:_____

Carbohydrate:_____

<u>Daily Energy Intake:</u>_____

Notes:_____

_____

_____

WEDNESDAY

Date:_____

Breakfast:

Time:_____

ate:_____

_____

_____

drank:_____

_____

Protein:_____ Fat:_____

Carbohydrate:_____

Snack:

Time:_____

_____

_____

_____

Lunch:

Time:_____

ate:_____

_____

_____

drank:_____

_____

Protein:_____ Fat:_____

Carbohydrate:_____

<u>Snack:</u>   Time:_____

_____

_____

_____

<u>Dinner:</u>   Time:_____

ate:_____

_____

_____

drank:_____

_____

Protein:_____ Fat:_____

Carbohydrate:_____

<u>Daily Energy Intake:</u>_____

Notes:_____

_____

_____

THURSDAY   Date:_____

Breakfast: Time:_____

ate:_____

_____

_____

drank:_____

_____

Protein:_____ Fat:_____

Carbohydrate:_____

Snack: Time:_____

_____

_____

_____

Lunch: Time:_____

ate:_____

_____

_____

drank:_____

_____

Protein:_____ Fat:_____

Carbohydrate:_____

Snack: Time:_____

_____

_____

_____

Dinner: Time:_____

ate:_____

_____

_____

drank:_____

_____

Protein:_____ Fat:_____

Carbohydrate:_____

Daily Energy Intake:_____

Notes:_____

_____

_____

FRIDAY   Date:_____

Breakfast: Time:_____

ate:_____

_____

_____

drank:_____

_____

Protein:_____ Fat:_____

Carbohydrate:_____

Snack: Time:_____

_____

_____

_____

Lunch: Time:_____

ate:_____

_____

_____

drank:_____

_____

Protein:_____ Fat:_____

Carbohydrate:_____

<u>Snack:</u>   Time:_____

_____

_____

_____

<u>Dinner:</u>   Time:_____

ate:_____

_____

_____

drank:_____

_____

Protein:_____ Fat:_____

Carbohydrate:_____

<u>Daily Energy Intake:</u>_____

Notes:_____

_____

_____

SATURDAY Date:_____

Breakfast: Time:_____

ate:_____

_____

_____

drank:_____

_____

Protein:_____ Fat:_____

Carbohydrate:_____

Snack: Time:_____

_____

_____

_____

Lunch: Time:_____

ate:_____

_____

_____

drank:_____

_____

Protein:_____ Fat:_____

Carbohydrate:_____

<u>Snack:</u>   Time:_____

_____

_____

_____

<u>Dinner:</u>   Time:_____

ate:_____

_____

_____

drank:_____

_____

Protein:_____ Fat:_____

Carbohydrate:_____

<u>Daily Energy Intake:</u>_____

Notes:_____

_____

_____

SUNDAY   Date:_____

Breakfast: Time:_____

ate:_____

_____

_____

drank:_____

_____

Protein:_____ Fat:_____

Carbohydrate:_____

Snack: Time:_____

_____

_____

_____

Lunch: Time:_____

ate:_____

_____

_____

drank:_____

_____

Protein:_____ Fat:_____

Carbohydrate:_____

Snack: Time:_____

_____

_____

_____

Dinner: Time:_____

ate:_____

_____

_____

drank:_____

_____

Protein:_____ Fat:_____

Carbohydrate:_____

Daily Energy Intake:_____

Notes:_____

_____

_____

MONDAY   Date:_____

Breakfast: Time:_____

ate:_____

_____

_____

drank:_____

_____

Protein:_____ Fat:_____

Carbohydrate:_____

Snack: Time:_____

_____

_____

_____

Lunch: Time:_____

ate:_____

_____

_____

drank:_____

_____

Protein:_____ Fat:_____

Carbohydrate:_____

<u>Snack:</u>   Time:_____

_____

_____

_____

<u>Dinner:</u>   Time:_____

ate:_____

_____

_____

drank:_____

_____

Protein:_____ Fat:_____

Carbohydrate:_____

<u>Daily Energy Intake:</u>_____

Notes:_____

_____

_____

TUESDAY Date:_____

Breakfast: Time:_____

ate:_____

_____

_____

drank:_____

_____

Protein:_____ Fat:_____

Carbohydrate:_____

Snack: Time:_____

_____

_____

_____

Lunch: Time:_____

ate:_____

_____

_____

drank:_____

_____

Protein:_____ Fat:_____

Carbohydrate:_____

<u>Snack:</u>   Time:_____

_____

_____

_____

<u>Dinner:</u>   Time:_____

ate:_____

_____

_____

drank:_____

_____

Protein:_____ Fat:_____

Carbohydrate:_____

<u>Daily Energy Intake:</u>_____

Notes:_____

_____

_____

WEDNESDAY

Date:_____

Breakfast:

Time:_____

ate:_____

_____

_____

drank:_____

_____

Protein:_____ Fat:_____

Carbohydrate:_____

Snack:

Time:_____

_____

_____

_____

Lunch:

Time:_____

ate:_____

_____

_____

drank:_____

_____

Protein:_____ Fat:_____

Carbohydrate:_____

Snack: Time:_____

_____

_____

_____

Dinner: Time:_____

ate:_____

_____

_____

drank:_____

_____

Protein:_____ Fat:_____

Carbohydrate:_____

<u>Daily Energy Intake:</u>_____

Notes:_____

_____

_____

THURSDAY   Date:_____

Breakfast: Time:_____

ate:_____

_____

_____

drank:_____

_____

Protein:_____ Fat:_____

Carbohydrate:_____

Snack: Time:_____

_____

_____

_____

Lunch: Time:_____

ate:_____

_____

_____

drank:_____

_____

Protein:_____ Fat:_____

Carbohydrate:_____

<u>Snack:</u>   Time:_____

_____

_____

_____

<u>Dinner:</u>   Time:_____

ate:_____

_____

_____

drank:_____

_____

Protein:_____ Fat:_____

Carbohydrate:_____

<u>Daily Energy Intake:</u>_____

Notes:_____

_____

_____

FRIDAY   Date:_____

Breakfast: Time:_____

ate:_____

_____

_____

drank:_____

_____

Protein:_____ Fat:_____
Carbohydrate:_____

Snack: Time:_____

_____

_____

_____

Lunch: Time:_____

ate:_____

_____

_____

drank:_____

_____

Protein:_____ Fat:_____

Carbohydrate:_____

Snack: Time:_____

_____

_____

_____

Dinner: Time:_____

ate:_____

_____

_____

drank:_____

_____

Protein:_____ Fat:_____

Carbohydrate:_____

<u>Daily Energy Intake:</u>_____

Notes:_____

_____

_____

SATURDAY   Date:_____

Breakfast: Time:_____

ate:_____

_____

_____

drank:_____

_____

Protein:_____ Fat:_____

Carbohydrate:_____

Snack: Time:_____

_____

_____

_____

Lunch: Time:_____

ate:_____

_____

_____

drank:_____

_____

Protein:_____ Fat:_____

Carbohydrate:_____

Snack: Time:_____

_____

_____

_____

Dinner: Time:_____

ate:_____

_____

_____

drank:_____

_____

Protein:_____ Fat:_____

Carbohydrate:_____

Daily Energy Intake:_____

Notes:_____

_____

_____

SUNDAY   Date:_____

Breakfast: Time:_____

ate:_____

_____

_____

drank:_____

_____

Protein:_____ Fat:_____

Carbohydrate:_____

Snack: Time:_____

_____

_____

_____

Lunch: Time:_____

ate:_____

_____

_____

drank:_____

_____

Protein:_____ Fat:_____

Carbohydrate:_____

<u>Snack:</u>   Time:_____

_____

_____

_____

<u>Dinner:</u>   Time:_____

ate:_____

_____

_____

drank:_____

_____

Protein:_____ Fat:_____

Carbohydrate:_____

<u>Daily Energy Intake:</u>_____

Notes:_____

_____

_____

MONDAY

Date:_____

Breakfast:

Time:_____

ate:_____

_____

_____

drank:_____

_____

Protein:_____ Fat:_____

Carbohydrate:_____

Snack:

Time:_____

_____

_____

_____

Lunch:

Time:_____

ate:_____

_____

_____

drank:_____

_____

Protein:_____ Fat:_____

Carbohydrate:_____

Snack: Time:_____

_____

_____

_____

Dinner: Time:_____

ate:_____

_____

_____

drank:_____

_____

Protein:_____ Fat:_____

Carbohydrate:_____

Daily Energy Intake:_____

Notes:_____

_____

_____

TUESDAY Date:_____

Breakfast: Time:_____

ate:_____

_____

_____

drank:_____

_____

Protein:_____ Fat:_____

Carbohydrate:_____

Snack: Time:_____

_____

_____

_____

Lunch: Time:_____

ate:_____

_____

_____

drank:_____

_____

Protein:_____ Fat:_____

Carbohydrate:_____

Snack: Time:_____

_____

_____

_____

Dinner: Time:_____

ate:_____

_____

_____

drank:_____

_____

Protein:_____ Fat:_____

Carbohydrate:_____

Daily Energy Intake:_____

Notes:_____

_____

_____

WEDNESDAY Date:_____

Breakfast: Time:_____

ate:_____

_____

_____

drank:_____

_____

Protein:_____ Fat:_____

Carbohydrate:_____

Snack: Time:_____

_____

_____

_____

Lunch: Time:_____

ate:_____

_____

_____

drank:_____

_____

Protein:_____ Fat:_____

Carbohydrate:_____

<u>Snack:</u> Time:_____

_____

_____

_____

<u>Dinner:</u> Time:_____

ate:_____

_____

_____

drank:_____

_____

Protein:_____ Fat:_____

Carbohydrate:_____

<u>Daily Energy Intake:</u>_____

Notes:_____

_____

_____

THURSDAY

Date:_____

Breakfast:

Time:_____

ate:_____

_____

_____

drank:_____

_____

Protein:_____ Fat:_____

Carbohydrate:_____

Snack:

Time:_____

_____

_____

_____

Lunch:

Time:_____

ate:_____

_____

_____

drank:_____

_____

Protein:_____ Fat:_____

Carbohydrate:_____

Snack: Time:_____

_____

_____

_____

Dinner: Time:_____

ate:_____

_____

_____

drank:_____

_____

Protein:_____ Fat:_____

Carbohydrate:_____

<u>Daily Energy Intake:</u>_____

Notes:_____

_____

_____

FRIDAY   Date:_____

Breakfast: Time:_____

ate:_____

_____

_____

drank:_____

_____

Protein:_____ Fat:_____

Carbohydrate:_____

Snack: Time:_____

_____

_____

_____

Lunch: Time:_____

ate:_____

_____

_____

drank:_____

_____

Protein:_____ Fat:_____

Carbohydrate:_____

Snack: Time:_____

_____

_____

_____

Dinner: Time:_____

ate:_____

_____

_____

drank:_____

_____

Protein:_____ Fat:_____

Carbohydrate:_____

Daily Energy Intake:_____

Notes:_____

_____

_____

SATURDAY   Date:_____

Breakfast: Time:_____

ate:_____

_____

_____

drank:_____

_____

Protein:_____ Fat:_____

Carbohydrate:_____

Snack: Time:_____

_____

_____

_____

Lunch: Time:_____

ate:_____

_____

_____

drank:_____

_____

Protein:_____ Fat:_____

Carbohydrate:_____

Snack: Time:_____

_____

_____

_____

Dinner: Time:_____

ate:_____

_____

_____

drank:_____

_____

Protein:_____ Fat:_____

Carbohydrate:_____

Daily Energy Intake:_____

Notes:_____

_____

_____

SUNDAY   Date:_____

Breakfast: Time:_____

ate:_____

_____

_____

drank:_____

_____

Protein:_____ Fat:_____

Carbohydrate:_____

Snack: Time:_____

_____

_____

_____

Lunch: Time:_____

ate:_____

_____

_____

drank:_____

_____

Protein:_____ Fat:_____

Carbohydrate:_____

<u>Snack:</u>   Time:_____

_____

_____

_____

<u>Dinner:</u>   Time:_____

ate:_____

_____

_____

drank:_____

_____

Protein:_____ Fat:_____

Carbohydrate:_____

<u>Daily Energy Intake:</u>_____

Notes:_____

_____

_____

APPRAISAL

Date:_____

Weight:
after 4 weeks_____ now _____

Body Fat:
after 4 weeks_____ now _____

Circumference
Tight:
after 4 weeks_____ now _____

Hip:
after 4 weeks_____ now _____

Waist:
after 4 weeks_____ now _____

Upper Arm:
after 4 weeks_____ now _____

Total Daily Energy Expenditure:_____
Daily Energy Intake:_____

Things about my body that already changed:

1._____

2._____

3._____

_____

_____

Things about my nutrition that already changed:

1._____

2._____

3._____

_____

_____

Things I still want to change:

1._____

2._____

3._____

_____

_____

NOTES

NOTES

NOTES